Personal Info	
Name:	D
Address:	
Mobile Telephone:	
Home Telephone:	
Email:	
Blood Group:	
Weight:	
Height:	

Doctor's Information	
Name:	Medication:
Hospital Address:	
Mobile Telephone:	
Email:	

Emergency Contact	
Name:	Relationship:
Address:	
Mobile Telephone:	
Home Telephone:	
Email:	

Modern Simple Press @ Business Log Book Series

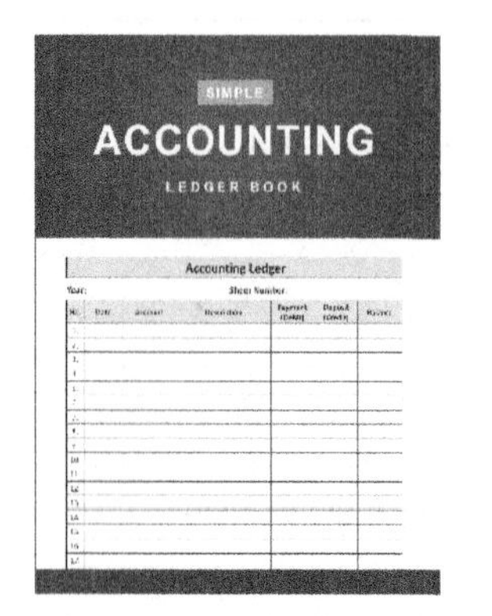

ASIN: B0943T8H1R

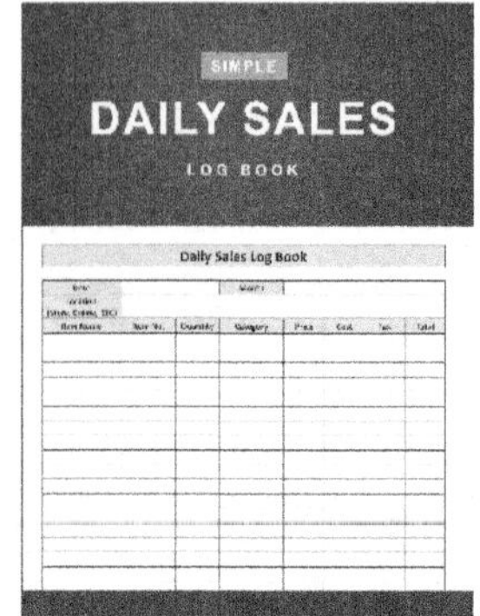

ASIN: B08XS7KYKC

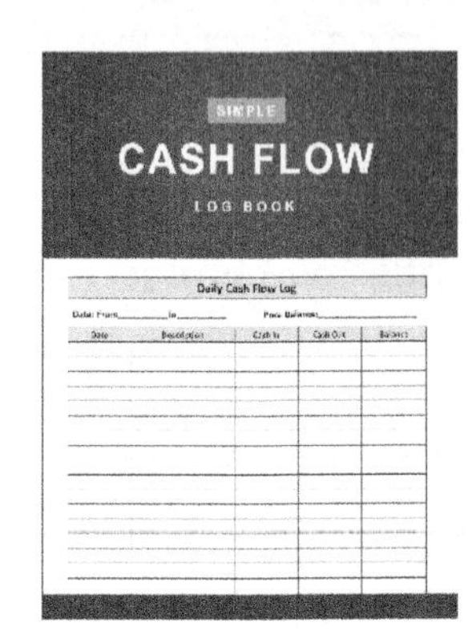

ASIN: B0914WWGNM

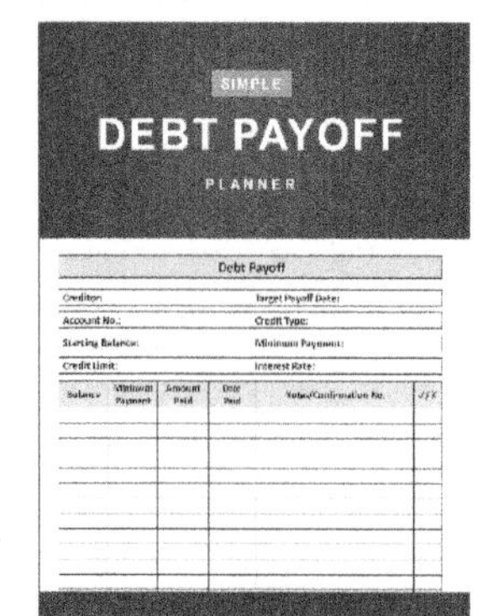

ASIN: B08MSQ3Z6Y

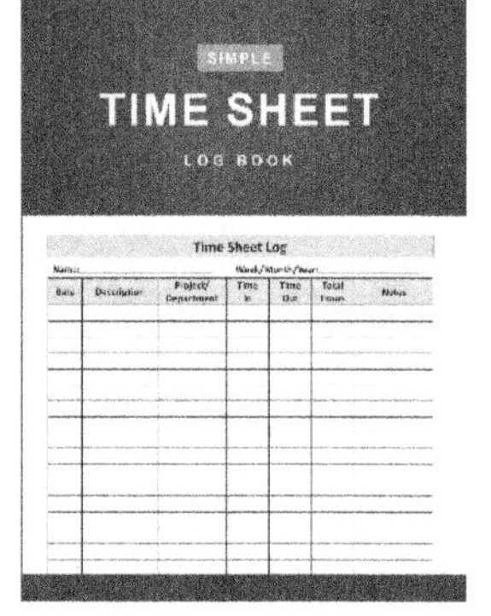

ASIN: B08MSKDJFS

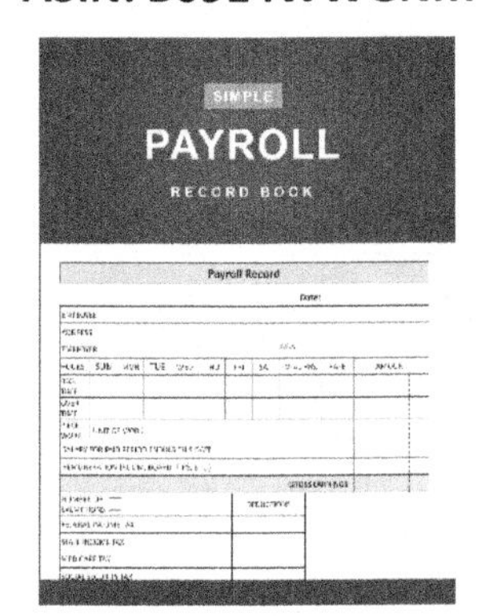

ASIN: B08MSQ3SGQ

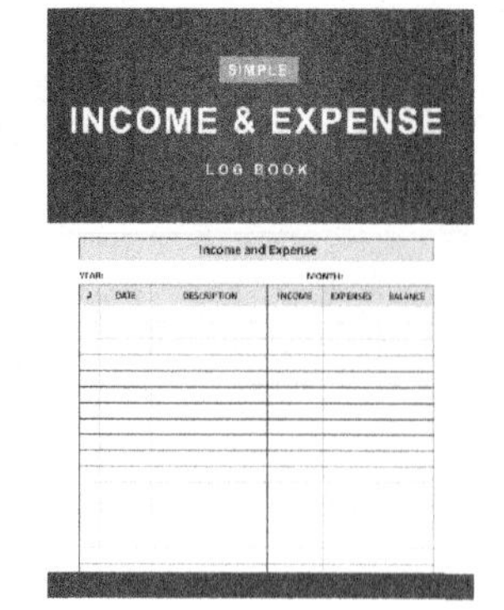

ASIN: B08LNBK4NZ

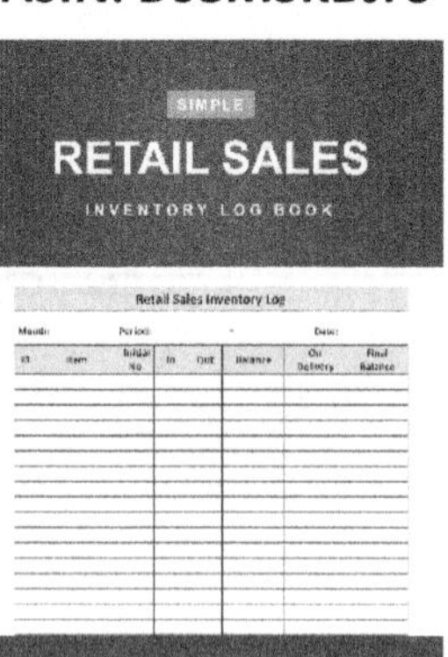

ASIN: B095GSG8VB

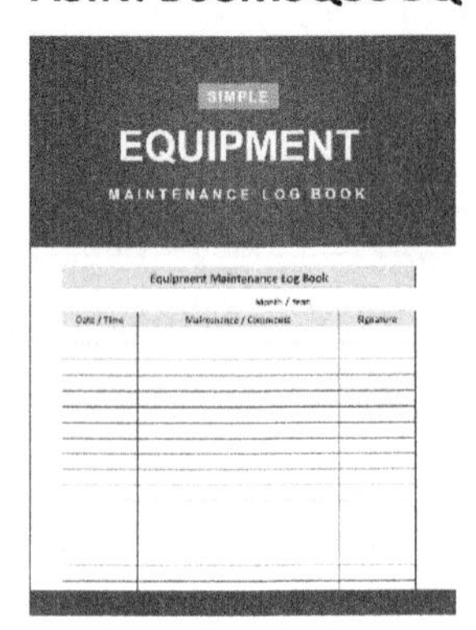

ASIN: B096J11TSJ

Modern Simple Press @ Freebies

We have a freebie for you!

Scan the QR Code
To get news, exclusive offers & free pages

Visit our Amazon author pages
@modernsimplepress

Blood Pressure Log

Month: ________________ **Week Starting:** __________________________

Time		Blood Pressure Systolic (upper #)	Blood Pressure Diastolic (lower #)	Heart Rate (pulse per minute)	Notes (e.g. medication changes, activities)
Monday	a.m.				
	a.m.				
	p.m.				
	p.m.				
Tuesday	a.m.				
	a.m.				
	p.m.				
	p.m.				
Wednesday	a.m.				
	a.m.				
	p.m.				
	p.m.				
Thursday	a.m.				
	a.m.				
	p.m.				
	p.m.				
Friday	a.m.				
	a.m.				
	p.m.				
	p.m.				
Saturday	a.m.				
	a.m.				
	p.m.				
	p.m.				
Sunday	a.m.				
	a.m.				
	p.m.				
	p.m.				

Blood Pressure Log

Month: ________________ Week Starting: _________________________

Time		Blood Pressure		Heart Rate (pulse per minute)	Notes (e.g. medication changes, activities)
		Systolic (upper #)	Diastolic (lower #)		
Monday	a.m.				
	a.m.				
	p.m.				
	p.m.				
Tuesday	a.m.				
	a.m.				
	p.m.				
	p.m.				
Wednesday	a.m.				
	a.m.				
	p.m.				
	p.m.				
Thursday	a.m.				
	a.m.				
	p.m.				
	p.m.				
Friday	a.m.				
	a.m.				
	p.m.				
	p.m.				
Saturday	a.m.				
	a.m.				
	p.m.				
	p.m.				
Sunday	a.m.				
	a.m.				
	p.m.				
	p.m.				

Blood Pressure Log

Month: ________________ **Week Starting:** __________________________

Time		Blood Pressure		Heart Rate (pulse per minute)	Notes (e.g. medication changes, activities)
		Systolic (upper #)	Diastolic (lower #)		
Monday	a.m.				
	a.m.				
	p.m.				
	p.m.				
Tuesday	a.m.				
	a.m.				
	p.m.				
	p.m.				
Wednesday	a.m.				
	a.m.				
	p.m.				
	p.m.				
Thursday	a.m.				
	a.m.				
	p.m.				
	p.m.				
Friday	a.m.				
	a.m.				
	p.m.				
	p.m.				
Saturday	a.m.				
	a.m.				
	p.m.				
	p.m.				
Sunday	a.m.				
	a.m.				
	p.m.				
	p.m.				

Blood Pressure Log

Month: ________________ Week Starting: ___________________________

Time		Blood Pressure		Heart Rate (pulse per minute)	Notes (e.g. medication changes, activities)
		Systolic (upper #)	Diastolic (lower #)		
Monday	a.m.				
	a.m.				
	p.m.				
	p.m.				
Tuesday	a.m.				
	a.m.				
	p.m.				
	p.m.				
Wednesday	a.m.				
	a.m.				
	p.m.				
	p.m.				
Thursday	a.m.				
	a.m.				
	p.m.				
	p.m.				
Friday	a.m.				
	a.m.				
	p.m.				
	p.m.				
Saturday	a.m.				
	a.m.				
	p.m.				
	p.m.				
Sunday	a.m.				
	a.m.				
	p.m.				
	p.m.				

Blood Pressure Log

Month: ________________ **Week Starting:** __________________________

Time		Blood Pressure		Heart Rate (pulse per minute)	Notes (e.g. medication changes, activities)
		Systolic (upper #)	Diastolic (lower #)		
Monday	a.m.				
	a.m.				
	p.m.				
	p.m.				
Tuesday	a.m.				
	a.m.				
	p.m.				
	p.m.				
Wednesday	a.m.				
	a.m.				
	p.m.				
	p.m.				
Thursday	a.m.				
	a.m.				
	p.m.				
	p.m.				
Friday	a.m.				
	a.m.				
	p.m.				
	p.m.				
Saturday	a.m.				
	a.m.				
	p.m.				
	p.m.				
Sunday	a.m.				
	a.m.				
	p.m.				
	p.m.				

Blood Pressure Log

Month: ________________ **Week Starting**: __________________________

Time		Blood Pressure Systolic (upper #)	Blood Pressure Diastolic (lower #)	Heart Rate (pulse per minute)	Notes (e.g. medication changes, activities)
Monday	a.m.				
	a.m.				
	p.m.				
	p.m.				
Tuesday	a.m.				
	a.m.				
	p.m.				
	p.m.				
Wednesday	a.m.				
	a.m.				
	p.m.				
	p.m.				
Thursday	a.m.				
	a.m.				
	p.m.				
	p.m.				
Friday	a.m.				
	a.m.				
	p.m.				
	p.m.				
Saturday	a.m.				
	a.m.				
	p.m.				
	p.m.				
Sunday	a.m.				
	a.m.				
	p.m.				
	p.m.				

Blood Pressure Log

Month: ________________ Week Starting: ___________________________

Time		Blood Pressure		Heart Rate (pulse per minute)	Notes (e.g. medication changes, activities)
		Systolic (upper #)	Diastolic (lower #)		
Monday	a.m.				
	a.m.				
	p.m.				
	p.m.				
Tuesday	a.m.				
	a.m.				
	p.m.				
	p.m.				
Wednesday	a.m.				
	a.m.				
	p.m.				
	p.m.				
Thursday	a.m.				
	a.m.				
	p.m.				
	p.m.				
Friday	a.m.				
	a.m.				
	p.m.				
	p.m.				
Saturday	a.m.				
	a.m.				
	p.m.				
	p.m.				
Sunday	a.m.				
	a.m.				
	p.m.				
	p.m.				

Blood Pressure Log

Month: ________________ **Week Starting:** _________________________

Time		Blood Pressure: Systolic (upper #)	Blood Pressure: Diastolic (lower #)	Heart Rate (pulse per minute)	Notes (e.g. medication changes, activities)
Monday	a.m.				
	a.m.				
	p.m.				
	p.m.				
Tuesday	a.m.				
	a.m.				
	p.m.				
	p.m.				
Wednesday	a.m.				
	a.m.				
	p.m.				
	p.m.				
Thursday	a.m.				
	a.m.				
	p.m.				
	p.m.				
Friday	a.m.				
	a.m.				
	p.m.				
	p.m.				
Saturday	a.m.				
	a.m.				
	p.m.				
	p.m.				
Sunday	a.m.				
	a.m.				
	p.m.				
	p.m.				

Blood Pressure Log

Month: ________________ **Week Starting:** ____________________________

Time		Blood Pressure		Heart Rate (pulse per minute)	Notes (e.g. medication changes, activities)
		Systolic (upper #)	Diastolic (lower #)		
Monday	a.m.				
	a.m.				
	p.m.				
	p.m.				
Tuesday	a.m.				
	a.m.				
	p.m.				
	p.m.				
Wednesday	a.m.				
	a.m.				
	p.m.				
	p.m.				
Thursday	a.m.				
	a.m.				
	p.m.				
	p.m.				
Friday	a.m.				
	a.m.				
	p.m.				
	p.m.				
Saturday	a.m.				
	a.m.				
	p.m.				
	p.m.				
Sunday	a.m.				
	a.m.				
	p.m.				
	p.m.				

Blood Pressure Log

Month: ________________ **Week Starting:** ____________________________

Time		Blood Pressure		Heart Rate (pulse per minute)	Notes (e.g. medication changes, activities)
		Systolic (upper #)	Diastolic (lower #)		
Monday	a.m.				
	a.m.				
	p.m.				
	p.m.				
Tuesday	a.m.				
	a.m.				
	p.m.				
	p.m.				
Wednesday	a.m.				
	a.m.				
	p.m.				
	p.m.				
Thursday	a.m.				
	a.m.				
	p.m.				
	p.m.				
Friday	a.m.				
	a.m.				
	p.m.				
	p.m.				
Saturday	a.m.				
	a.m.				
	p.m.				
	p.m.				
Sunday	a.m.				
	a.m.				
	p.m.				
	p.m.				

Blood Pressure Log					

Month: _______________ Week Starting: ________________________

Time		Blood Pressure		Heart Rate (pulse per minute)	Notes (e.g. medication changes, activities)
		Systolic (upper #)	Diastolic (lower #)		
Monday	a.m.				
	a.m.				
	p.m.				
	p.m.				
Tuesday	a.m.				
	a.m.				
	p.m.				
	p.m.				
Wednesday	a.m.				
	a.m.				
	p.m.				
	p.m.				
Thursday	a.m.				
	a.m.				
	p.m.				
	p.m.				
Friday	a.m.				
	a.m.				
	p.m.				
	p.m.				
Saturday	a.m.				
	a.m.				
	p.m.				
	p.m.				
Sunday	a.m.				
	a.m.				
	p.m.				
	p.m.				

Blood Pressure Log

Month: ________________ Week Starting: ________________________

Time		Blood Pressure		Heart Rate (pulse per minute)	Notes (e.g. medication changes, activities)
		Systolic (upper #)	Diastolic (lower #)		
Monday	a.m.				
	a.m.				
	p.m.				
	p.m.				
Tuesday	a.m.				
	a.m.				
	p.m.				
	p.m.				
Wednesday	a.m.				
	a.m.				
	p.m.				
	p.m.				
Thursday	a.m.				
	a.m.				
	p.m.				
	p.m.				
Friday	a.m.				
	a.m.				
	p.m.				
	p.m.				
Saturday	a.m.				
	a.m.				
	p.m.				
	p.m.				
Sunday	a.m.				
	a.m.				
	p.m.				
	p.m.				

Blood Pressure Log

Month: ________________ **Week Starting:** __________________________

Time		Blood Pressure		Heart Rate (pulse per minute)	Notes (e.g. medication changes, activities)
		Systolic (upper #)	Diastolic (lower #)		
Monday	a.m.				
	a.m.				
	p.m.				
	p.m.				
Tuesday	a.m.				
	a.m.				
	p.m.				
	p.m.				
Wednesday	a.m.				
	a.m.				
	p.m.				
	p.m.				
Thursday	a.m.				
	a.m.				
	p.m.				
	p.m.				
Friday	a.m.				
	a.m.				
	p.m.				
	p.m.				
Saturday	a.m.				
	a.m.				
	p.m.				
	p.m.				
Sunday	a.m.				
	a.m.				
	p.m.				
	p.m.				

Blood Pressure Log

Month: ________________ Week Starting: _________________________

Time		Blood Pressure		Heart Rate (pulse per minute)	Notes (e.g. medication changes, activities)
		Systolic (upper #)	Diastolic (lower #)		
Monday	a.m.				
	a.m.				
	p.m.				
	p.m.				
Tuesday	a.m.				
	a.m.				
	p.m.				
	p.m.				
Wednesday	a.m.				
	a.m.				
	p.m.				
	p.m.				
Thursday	a.m.				
	a.m.				
	p.m.				
	p.m.				
Friday	a.m.				
	a.m.				
	p.m.				
	p.m.				
Saturday	a.m.				
	a.m.				
	p.m.				
	p.m.				
Sunday	a.m.				
	a.m.				
	p.m.				
	p.m.				

Blood Pressure Log

Month: ______________ **Week Starting:** ______________________

Time		Blood Pressure		Heart Rate (pulse per minute)	Notes (e.g. medication changes, activities)
		Systolic (upper #)	Diastolic (lower #)		
Monday	a.m.				
	a.m.				
	p.m.				
	p.m.				
Tuesday	a.m.				
	a.m.				
	p.m.				
	p.m.				
Wednesday	a.m.				
	a.m.				
	p.m.				
	p.m.				
Thursday	a.m.				
	a.m.				
	p.m.				
	p.m.				
Friday	a.m.				
	a.m.				
	p.m.				
	p.m.				
Saturday	a.m.				
	a.m.				
	p.m.				
	p.m.				
Sunday	a.m.				
	a.m.				
	p.m.				
	p.m.				

Blood Pressure Log

Month: ________________ **Week Starting:** _________________________

Time		Blood Pressure		Heart Rate (pulse per minute)	Notes (e.g. medication changes, activities)
		Systolic (upper #)	Diastolic (lower #)		
Monday	a.m.				
	a.m.				
	p.m.				
	p.m.				
Tuesday	a.m.				
	a.m.				
	p.m.				
	p.m.				
Wednesday	a.m.				
	a.m.				
	p.m.				
	p.m.				
Thursday	a.m.				
	a.m.				
	p.m.				
	p.m.				
Friday	a.m.				
	a.m.				
	p.m.				
	p.m.				
Saturday	a.m.				
	a.m.				
	p.m.				
	p.m.				
Sunday	a.m.				
	a.m.				
	p.m.				
	p.m.				

Blood Pressure Log

Month: ________________ **Week Starting:** ____________________________

Time		Blood Pressure: Systolic (upper #)	Blood Pressure: Diastolic (lower #)	Heart Rate (pulse per minute)	Notes (e.g. medication changes, activities)
Monday	a.m.				
	a.m.				
	p.m.				
	p.m.				
Tuesday	a.m.				
	a.m.				
	p.m.				
	p.m.				
Wednesday	a.m.				
	a.m.				
	p.m.				
	p.m.				
Thursday	a.m.				
	a.m.				
	p.m.				
	p.m.				
Friday	a.m.				
	a.m.				
	p.m.				
	p.m.				
Saturday	a.m.				
	a.m.				
	p.m.				
	p.m.				
Sunday	a.m.				
	a.m.				
	p.m.				
	p.m.				

Blood Pressure Log

Month: ________________ **Week Starting:** __________________________

Time		Blood Pressure		Heart Rate (pulse per minute)	Notes (e.g. medication changes, activities)
		Systolic (upper #)	Diastolic (lower #)		
Monday	a.m.				
	a.m.				
	p.m.				
	p.m.				
Tuesday	a.m.				
	a.m.				
	p.m.				
	p.m.				
Wednesday	a.m.				
	a.m.				
	p.m.				
	p.m.				
Thursday	a.m.				
	a.m.				
	p.m.				
	p.m.				
Friday	a.m.				
	a.m.				
	p.m.				
	p.m.				
Saturday	a.m.				
	a.m.				
	p.m.				
	p.m.				
Sunday	a.m.				
	a.m.				
	p.m.				
	p.m.				

Blood Pressure Log

Month: ______________ **Week Starting:** ______________________

Time		Blood Pressure		Heart Rate (pulse per minute)	Notes (e.g. medication changes, activities)
		Systolic (upper #)	Diastolic (lower #)		
Monday	a.m.				
	a.m.				
	p.m.				
	p.m.				
Tuesday	a.m.				
	a.m.				
	p.m.				
	p.m.				
Wednesday	a.m.				
	a.m.				
	p.m.				
	p.m.				
Thursday	a.m.				
	a.m.				
	p.m.				
	p.m.				
Friday	a.m.				
	a.m.				
	p.m.				
	p.m.				
Saturday	a.m.				
	a.m.				
	p.m.				
	p.m.				
Sunday	a.m.				
	a.m.				
	p.m.				
	p.m.				

Blood Pressure Log

Month: ________________ Week Starting: _________________________

Time		Blood Pressure		Heart Rate (pulse per minute)	Notes (e.g. medication changes, activities)
		Systolic (upper #)	Diastolic (lower #)		
Monday	a.m.				
	a.m.				
	p.m.				
	p.m.				
Tuesday	a.m.				
	a.m.				
	p.m.				
	p.m.				
Wednesday	a.m.				
	a.m.				
	p.m.				
	p.m.				
Thursday	a.m.				
	a.m.				
	p.m.				
	p.m.				
Friday	a.m.				
	a.m.				
	p.m.				
	p.m.				
Saturday	a.m.				
	a.m.				
	p.m.				
	p.m.				
Sunday	a.m.				
	a.m.				
	p.m.				
	p.m.				

Blood Pressure Log

Month: ______________ Week Starting: ______________________

Time		Blood Pressure		Heart Rate (pulse per minute)	Notes (e.g. medication changes, activities)
		Systolic (upper #)	Diastolic (lower #)		
Monday	a.m.				
	a.m.				
	p.m.				
	p.m.				
Tuesday	a.m.				
	a.m.				
	p.m.				
	p.m.				
Wednesday	a.m.				
	a.m.				
	p.m.				
	p.m.				
Thursday	a.m.				
	a.m.				
	p.m.				
	p.m.				
Friday	a.m.				
	a.m.				
	p.m.				
	p.m.				
Saturday	a.m.				
	a.m.				
	p.m.				
	p.m.				
Sunday	a.m.				
	a.m.				
	p.m.				
	p.m.				

Blood Pressure Log

Month: ________________ Week Starting: ______________________

Time		Blood Pressure		Heart Rate (pulse per minute)	Notes (e.g. medication changes, activities)
		Systolic (upper #)	Diastolic (lower #)		
Monday	a.m.				
	a.m.				
	p.m.				
	p.m.				
Tuesday	a.m.				
	a.m.				
	p.m.				
	p.m.				
Wednesday	a.m.				
	a.m.				
	p.m.				
	p.m.				
Thursday	a.m.				
	a.m.				
	p.m.				
	p.m.				
Friday	a.m.				
	a.m.				
	p.m.				
	p.m.				
Saturday	a.m.				
	a.m.				
	p.m.				
	p.m.				
Sunday	a.m.				
	a.m.				
	p.m.				
	p.m.				

Blood Pressure Log

Month: ______________ Week Starting: ______________________

Time		Blood Pressure		Heart Rate (pulse per minute)	Notes (e.g. medication changes, activities)
		Systolic (upper #)	Diastolic (lower #)		
Monday	a.m.				
	a.m.				
	p.m.				
	p.m.				
Tuesday	a.m.				
	a.m.				
	p.m.				
	p.m.				
Wednesday	a.m.				
	a.m.				
	p.m.				
	p.m.				
Thursday	a.m.				
	a.m.				
	p.m.				
	p.m.				
Friday	a.m.				
	a.m.				
	p.m.				
	p.m.				
Saturday	a.m.				
	a.m.				
	p.m.				
	p.m.				
Sunday	a.m.				
	a.m.				
	p.m.				
	p.m.				

Blood Pressure Log

Month: ________________ **Week Starting:** __________________________

Time		Blood Pressure		Heart Rate (pulse per minute)	Notes (e.g. medication changes, activities)
		Systolic (upper #)	Diastolic (lower #)		
Monday	a.m.				
	a.m.				
	p.m.				
	p.m.				
Tuesday	a.m.				
	a.m.				
	p.m.				
	p.m.				
Wednesday	a.m.				
	a.m.				
	p.m.				
	p.m.				
Thursday	a.m.				
	a.m.				
	p.m.				
	p.m.				
Friday	a.m.				
	a.m.				
	p.m.				
	p.m.				
Saturday	a.m.				
	a.m.				
	p.m.				
	p.m.				
Sunday	a.m.				
	a.m.				
	p.m.				
	p.m.				

Blood Pressure Log					

Month: ______________ Week Starting: ______________________

Time		Blood Pressure		Heart Rate (pulse per minute)	Notes (e.g. medication changes, activities)
		Systolic (upper #)	Diastolic (lower #)		
Monday	a.m.				
	a.m.				
	p.m.				
	p.m.				
Tuesday	a.m.				
	a.m.				
	p.m.				
	p.m.				
Wednesday	a.m.				
	a.m.				
	p.m.				
	p.m.				
Thursday	a.m.				
	a.m.				
	p.m.				
	p.m.				
Friday	a.m.				
	a.m.				
	p.m.				
	p.m.				
Saturday	a.m.				
	a.m.				
	p.m.				
	p.m.				
Sunday	a.m.				
	a.m.				
	p.m.				
	p.m.				

Blood Pressure Log

Month: ________________ Week Starting: ___________________________

Time		Blood Pressure		Heart Rate (pulse per minute)	Notes (e.g. medication changes, activities)
		Systolic (upper #)	Diastolic (lower #)		
Monday	a.m.				
	a.m.				
	p.m.				
	p.m.				
Tuesday	a.m.				
	a.m.				
	p.m.				
	p.m.				
Wednesday	a.m.				
	a.m.				
	p.m.				
	p.m.				
Thursday	a.m.				
	a.m.				
	p.m.				
	p.m.				
Friday	a.m.				
	a.m.				
	p.m.				
	p.m.				
Saturday	a.m.				
	a.m.				
	p.m.				
	p.m.				
Sunday	a.m.				
	a.m.				
	p.m.				
	p.m.				

Blood Pressure Log

Month: ________________ Week Starting: __________________________

Time		Blood Pressure		Heart Rate (pulse per minute)	Notes (e.g. medication changes, activities)
		Systolic (upper #)	Diastolic (lower #)		
Monday	a.m.				
	a.m.				
	p.m.				
	p.m.				
Tuesday	a.m.				
	a.m.				
	p.m.				
	p.m.				
Wednesday	a.m.				
	a.m.				
	p.m.				
	p.m.				
Thursday	a.m.				
	a.m.				
	p.m.				
	p.m.				
Friday	a.m.				
	a.m.				
	p.m.				
	p.m.				
Saturday	a.m.				
	a.m.				
	p.m.				
	p.m.				
Sunday	a.m.				
	a.m.				
	p.m.				
	p.m.				

Blood Pressure Log

Month: ________________ **Week Starting:** _________________________

Time		Blood Pressure Systolic (upper #)	Diastolic (lower #)	Heart Rate (pulse per minute)	Notes (e.g. medication changes, activities)
Monday	a.m.				
	a.m.				
	p.m.				
	p.m.				
Tuesday	a.m.				
	a.m.				
	p.m.				
	p.m.				
Wednesday	a.m.				
	a.m.				
	p.m.				
	p.m.				
Thursday	a.m.				
	a.m.				
	p.m.				
	p.m.				
Friday	a.m.				
	a.m.				
	p.m.				
	p.m.				
Saturday	a.m.				
	a.m.				
	p.m.				
	p.m.				
Sunday	a.m.				
	a.m.				
	p.m.				
	p.m.				

Blood Pressure Log

Month: _______________ Week Starting: _______________________

Time		Blood Pressure		Heart Rate (pulse per minute)	Notes (e.g. medication changes, activities)
		Systolic (upper #)	Diastolic (lower #)		
Monday	a.m.				
	a.m.				
	p.m.				
	p.m.				
Tuesday	a.m.				
	a.m.				
	p.m.				
	p.m.				
Wednesday	a.m.				
	a.m.				
	p.m.				
	p.m.				
Thursday	a.m.				
	a.m.				
	p.m.				
	p.m.				
Friday	a.m.				
	a.m.				
	p.m.				
	p.m.				
Saturday	a.m.				
	a.m.				
	p.m.				
	p.m.				
Sunday	a.m.				
	a.m.				
	p.m.				
	p.m.				

Blood Pressure Log

Month: _______________ **Week Starting:** _______________________

Time		Blood Pressure		Heart Rate (pulse per minute)	Notes (e.g. medication changes, activities)
		Systolic (upper #)	**Diastolic** (lower #)		
Monday	a.m.				
	a.m.				
	p.m.				
	p.m.				
Tuesday	a.m.				
	a.m.				
	p.m.				
	p.m.				
Wednesday	a.m.				
	a.m.				
	p.m.				
	p.m.				
Thursday	a.m.				
	a.m.				
	p.m.				
	p.m.				
Friday	a.m.				
	a.m.				
	p.m.				
	p.m.				
Saturday	a.m.				
	a.m.				
	p.m.				
	p.m.				
Sunday	a.m.				
	a.m.				
	p.m.				
	p.m.				

Blood Pressure Log

Month: ________________ **Week Starting:** __________________________

Time		Blood Pressure		Heart Rate (pulse per minute)	Notes (e.g. medication changes, activities)
		Systolic (upper #)	Diastolic (lower #)		
Monday	a.m.				
	a.m.				
	p.m.				
	p.m.				
Tuesday	a.m.				
	a.m.				
	p.m.				
	p.m.				
Wednesday	a.m.				
	a.m.				
	p.m.				
	p.m.				
Thursday	a.m.				
	a.m.				
	p.m.				
	p.m.				
Friday	a.m.				
	a.m.				
	p.m.				
	p.m.				
Saturday	a.m.				
	a.m.				
	p.m.				
	p.m.				
Sunday	a.m.				
	a.m.				
	p.m.				
	p.m.				

Blood Pressure Log

Month: ________________ Week Starting: __________________________

Time		Blood Pressure		Heart Rate (pulse per minute)	Notes (e.g. medication changes, activities)
		Systolic (upper #)	Diastolic (lower #)		
Monday	a.m.				
	a.m.				
	p.m.				
	p.m.				
Tuesday	a.m.				
	a.m.				
	p.m.				
	p.m.				
Wednesday	a.m.				
	a.m.				
	p.m.				
	p.m.				
Thursday	a.m.				
	a.m.				
	p.m.				
	p.m.				
Friday	a.m.				
	a.m.				
	p.m.				
	p.m.				
Saturday	a.m.				
	a.m.				
	p.m.				
	p.m.				
Sunday	a.m.				
	a.m.				
	p.m.				
	p.m.				

Blood Pressure Log

Month: ________________ **Week Starting:** __________________________

Time		Blood Pressure		Heart Rate (pulse per minute)	Notes (e.g. medication changes, activities)
		Systolic (upper #)	**Diastolic** (lower #)		
Monday	a.m.				
	a.m.				
	p.m.				
	p.m.				
Tuesday	a.m.				
	a.m.				
	p.m.				
	p.m.				
Wednesday	a.m.				
	a.m.				
	p.m.				
	p.m.				
Thursday	a.m.				
	a.m.				
	p.m.				
	p.m.				
Friday	a.m.				
	a.m.				
	p.m.				
	p.m.				
Saturday	a.m.				
	a.m.				
	p.m.				
	p.m.				
Sunday	a.m.				
	a.m.				
	p.m.				
	p.m.				

Blood Pressure Log

Month: ________________ **Week Starting:** ________________________

Time		Blood Pressure		Heart Rate (pulse per minute)	Notes (e.g. medication changes, activities)
		Systolic (upper #)	Diastolic (lower #)		
Monday	a.m.				
	a.m.				
	p.m.				
	p.m.				
Tuesday	a.m.				
	a.m.				
	p.m.				
	p.m.				
Wednesday	a.m.				
	a.m.				
	p.m.				
	p.m.				
Thursday	a.m.				
	a.m.				
	p.m.				
	p.m.				
Friday	a.m.				
	a.m.				
	p.m.				
	p.m.				
Saturday	a.m.				
	a.m.				
	p.m.				
	p.m.				
Sunday	a.m.				
	a.m.				
	p.m.				
	p.m.				

Blood Pressure Log

Month: ________________ **Week Starting:** ____________________________

Time		Blood Pressure		Heart Rate (pulse per minute)	Notes (e.g. medication changes, activities)
		Systolic (upper #)	Diastolic (lower #)		
Monday	a.m.				
	a.m.				
	p.m.				
	p.m.				
Tuesday	a.m.				
	a.m.				
	p.m.				
	p.m.				
Wednesday	a.m.				
	a.m.				
	p.m.				
	p.m.				
Thursday	a.m.				
	a.m.				
	p.m.				
	p.m.				
Friday	a.m.				
	a.m.				
	p.m.				
	p.m.				
Saturday	a.m.				
	a.m.				
	p.m.				
	p.m.				
Sunday	a.m.				
	a.m.				
	p.m.				
	p.m.				

Blood Pressure Log

Month: ______________ Week Starting: ______________________

Time		Blood Pressure		Heart Rate (pulse per minute)	Notes (e.g. medication changes, activities)
		Systolic (upper #)	Diastolic (lower #)		
Monday	a.m.				
	a.m.				
	p.m.				
	p.m.				
Tuesday	a.m.				
	a.m.				
	p.m.				
	p.m.				
Wednesday	a.m.				
	a.m.				
	p.m.				
	p.m.				
Thursday	a.m.				
	a.m.				
	p.m.				
	p.m.				
Friday	a.m.				
	a.m.				
	p.m.				
	p.m.				
Saturday	a.m.				
	a.m.				
	p.m.				
	p.m.				
Sunday	a.m.				
	a.m.				
	p.m.				
	p.m.				

Blood Pressure Log

Month: ______________ **Week Starting:** ________________________

Time		Blood Pressure		Heart Rate (pulse per minute)	Notes (e.g. medication changes, activities)
		Systolic (upper #)	Diastolic (lower #)		
Monday	a.m.				
	a.m.				
	p.m.				
	p.m.				
Tuesday	a.m.				
	a.m.				
	p.m.				
	p.m.				
Wednesday	a.m.				
	a.m.				
	p.m.				
	p.m.				
Thursday	a.m.				
	a.m.				
	p.m.				
	p.m.				
Friday	a.m.				
	a.m.				
	p.m.				
	p.m.				
Saturday	a.m.				
	a.m.				
	p.m.				
	p.m.				
Sunday	a.m.				
	a.m.				
	p.m.				
	p.m.				

Blood Pressure Log

Month: ________________ **Week Starting:** ________________________

Time		Blood Pressure Systolic (upper #)	Blood Pressure Diastolic (lower #)	Heart Rate (pulse per minute)	Notes (e.g. medication changes, activities)
Monday	a.m.				
	a.m.				
	p.m.				
	p.m.				
Tuesday	a.m.				
	a.m.				
	p.m.				
	p.m.				
Wednesday	a.m.				
	a.m.				
	p.m.				
	p.m.				
Thursday	a.m.				
	a.m.				
	p.m.				
	p.m.				
Friday	a.m.				
	a.m.				
	p.m.				
	p.m.				
Saturday	a.m.				
	a.m.				
	p.m.				
	p.m.				
Sunday	a.m.				
	a.m.				
	p.m.				
	p.m.				

Blood Pressure Log

Month: ________________ **Week Starting:** ________________________

Time		Blood Pressure		Heart Rate (pulse per minute)	Notes (e.g. medication changes, activities)
		Systolic (upper #)	**Diastolic** (lower #)		
Monday	a.m.				
	a.m.				
	p.m.				
	p.m.				
Tuesday	a.m.				
	a.m.				
	p.m.				
	p.m.				
Wednesday	a.m.				
	a.m.				
	p.m.				
	p.m.				
Thursday	a.m.				
	a.m.				
	p.m.				
	p.m.				
Friday	a.m.				
	a.m.				
	p.m.				
	p.m.				
Saturday	a.m.				
	a.m.				
	p.m.				
	p.m.				
Sunday	a.m.				
	a.m.				
	p.m.				
	p.m.				

Blood Pressure Log

Month: ________________ **Week Starting:** _________________________

Time		Blood Pressure Systolic (upper #)	Diastolic (lower #)	Heart Rate (pulse per minute)	Notes (e.g. medication changes, activities)
Monday	a.m.				
	a.m.				
	p.m.				
	p.m.				
Tuesday	a.m.				
	a.m.				
	p.m.				
	p.m.				
Wednesday	a.m.				
	a.m.				
	p.m.				
	p.m.				
Thursday	a.m.				
	a.m.				
	p.m.				
	p.m.				
Friday	a.m.				
	a.m.				
	p.m.				
	p.m.				
Saturday	a.m.				
	a.m.				
	p.m.				
	p.m.				
Sunday	a.m.				
	a.m.				
	p.m.				
	p.m.				

Blood Pressure Log

Month: ________________ **Week Starting:** __________________________

Time		**Blood Pressure**		**Heart Rate** (pulse per minute)	**Notes** (e.g. medication changes, activities)
		Systolic (upper #)	**Diastolic** (lower #)		
Monday	a.m.				
	a.m.				
	p.m.				
	p.m.				
Tuesday	a.m.				
	a.m.				
	p.m.				
	p.m.				
Wednesday	a.m.				
	a.m.				
	p.m.				
	p.m.				
Thursday	a.m.				
	a.m.				
	p.m.				
	p.m.				
Friday	a.m.				
	a.m.				
	p.m.				
	p.m.				
Saturday	a.m.				
	a.m.				
	p.m.				
	p.m.				
Sunday	a.m.				
	a.m.				
	p.m.				
	p.m.				

Blood Pressure Log

Month: ________________ **Week Starting:** ________________________

Time		Blood Pressure		Heart Rate (pulse per minute)	Notes (e.g. medication changes, activities)
		Systolic (upper #)	Diastolic (lower #)		
Monday	a.m.				
	a.m.				
	p.m.				
	p.m.				
Tuesday	a.m.				
	a.m.				
	p.m.				
	p.m.				
Wednesday	a.m.				
	a.m.				
	p.m.				
	p.m.				
Thursday	a.m.				
	a.m.				
	p.m.				
	p.m.				
Friday	a.m.				
	a.m.				
	p.m.				
	p.m.				
Saturday	a.m.				
	a.m.				
	p.m.				
	p.m.				
Sunday	a.m.				
	a.m.				
	p.m.				
	p.m.				

Blood Pressure Log

Month: ________________ **Week Starting:** _________________________

Time		**Blood Pressure**		**Heart Rate** (pulse per minute)	**Notes** (e.g. medication changes, activities)
		Systolic (upper #)	**Diastolic** (lower #)		
Monday	a.m.				
	a.m.				
	p.m.				
	p.m.				
Tuesday	a.m.				
	a.m.				
	p.m.				
	p.m.				
Wednesday	a.m.				
	a.m.				
	p.m.				
	p.m.				
Thursday	a.m.				
	a.m.				
	p.m.				
	p.m.				
Friday	a.m.				
	a.m.				
	p.m.				
	p.m.				
Saturday	a.m.				
	a.m.				
	p.m.				
	p.m.				
Sunday	a.m.				
	a.m.				
	p.m.				
	p.m.				

Blood Pressure Log

Month: ________________ Week Starting: _________________________

Time		Blood Pressure		Heart Rate (pulse per minute)	Notes (e.g. medication changes, activities)
		Systolic (upper #)	Diastolic (lower #)		
Monday	a.m.				
	a.m.				
	p.m.				
	p.m.				
Tuesday	a.m.				
	a.m.				
	p.m.				
	p.m.				
Wednesday	a.m.				
	a.m.				
	p.m.				
	p.m.				
Thursday	a.m.				
	a.m.				
	p.m.				
	p.m.				
Friday	a.m.				
	a.m.				
	p.m.				
	p.m.				
Saturday	a.m.				
	a.m.				
	p.m.				
	p.m.				
Sunday	a.m.				
	a.m.				
	p.m.				
	p.m.				

Blood Pressure Log

Month: ________________ Week Starting: ____________________________

Time		Blood Pressure		Heart Rate (pulse per minute)	Notes (e.g. medication changes, activities)
		Systolic (upper #)	Diastolic (lower #)		
Monday	a.m.				
	a.m.				
	p.m.				
	p.m.				
Tuesday	a.m.				
	a.m.				
	p.m.				
	p.m.				
Wednesday	a.m.				
	a.m.				
	p.m.				
	p.m.				
Thursday	a.m.				
	a.m.				
	p.m.				
	p.m.				
Friday	a.m.				
	a.m.				
	p.m.				
	p.m.				
Saturday	a.m.				
	a.m.				
	p.m.				
	p.m.				
Sunday	a.m.				
	a.m.				
	p.m.				
	p.m.				

Blood Pressure Log

Month: ________________ **Week Starting:** ________________________

Time		**Blood Pressure**		**Heart Rate** (pulse per minute)	**Notes** (e.g. medication changes, activities)
		Systolic (upper #)	**Diastolic** (lower #)		
Monday	a.m.				
	a.m.				
	p.m.				
	p.m.				
Tuesday	a.m.				
	a.m.				
	p.m.				
	p.m.				
Wednesday	a.m.				
	a.m.				
	p.m.				
	p.m.				
Thursday	a.m.				
	a.m.				
	p.m.				
	p.m.				
Friday	a.m.				
	a.m.				
	p.m.				
	p.m.				
Saturday	a.m.				
	a.m.				
	p.m.				
	p.m.				
Sunday	a.m.				
	a.m.				
	p.m.				
	p.m.				

Blood Pressure Log

Month: ________________ **Week Starting:** ______________________________

Time		Blood Pressure		Heart Rate (pulse per minute)	Notes (e.g. medication changes, activities)
		Systolic (upper #)	Diastolic (lower #)		
Monday	a.m.				
	a.m.				
	p.m.				
	p.m.				
Tuesday	a.m.				
	a.m.				
	p.m.				
	p.m.				
Wednesday	a.m.				
	a.m.				
	p.m.				
	p.m.				
Thursday	a.m.				
	a.m.				
	p.m.				
	p.m.				
Friday	a.m.				
	a.m.				
	p.m.				
	p.m.				
Saturday	a.m.				
	a.m.				
	p.m.				
	p.m.				
Sunday	a.m.				
	a.m.				
	p.m.				
	p.m.				

Blood Pressure Log

Month: ________________ **Week Starting:** __________________________

Time		Blood Pressure		Heart Rate (pulse per minute)	Notes (e.g. medication changes, activities)
		Systolic (upper #)	Diastolic (lower #)		
Monday	a.m.				
	a.m.				
	p.m.				
	p.m.				
Tuesday	a.m.				
	a.m.				
	p.m.				
	p.m.				
Wednesday	a.m.				
	a.m.				
	p.m.				
	p.m.				
Thursday	a.m.				
	a.m.				
	p.m.				
	p.m.				
Friday	a.m.				
	a.m.				
	p.m.				
	p.m.				
Saturday	a.m.				
	a.m.				
	p.m.				
	p.m.				
Sunday	a.m.				
	a.m.				
	p.m.				
	p.m.				

Blood Pressure Log

Month: ______________ **Week Starting:** ______________________

Time		Blood Pressure		Heart Rate (pulse per minute)	Notes (e.g. medication changes, activities)
		Systolic (upper #)	Diastolic (lower #)		
Monday	a.m.				
	a.m.				
	p.m.				
	p.m.				
Tuesday	a.m.				
	a.m.				
	p.m.				
	p.m.				
Wednesday	a.m.				
	a.m.				
	p.m.				
	p.m.				
Thursday	a.m.				
	a.m.				
	p.m.				
	p.m.				
Friday	a.m.				
	a.m.				
	p.m.				
	p.m.				
Saturday	a.m.				
	a.m.				
	p.m.				
	p.m.				
Sunday	a.m.				
	a.m.				
	p.m.				
	p.m.				

Blood Pressure Log

Month: ________________ **Week Starting:** ________________________

Time		Blood Pressure		Heart Rate (pulse per minute)	Notes (e.g. medication changes, activities)
		Systolic (upper #)	Diastolic (lower #)		
Monday	a.m.				
	a.m.				
	p.m.				
	p.m.				
Tuesday	a.m.				
	a.m.				
	p.m.				
	p.m.				
Wednesday	a.m.				
	a.m.				
	p.m.				
	p.m.				
Thursday	a.m.				
	a.m.				
	p.m.				
	p.m.				
Friday	a.m.				
	a.m.				
	p.m.				
	p.m.				
Saturday	a.m.				
	a.m.				
	p.m.				
	p.m.				
Sunday	a.m.				
	a.m.				
	p.m.				
	p.m.				

Blood Pressure Log

Month: ______________ Week Starting: ______________________

Time		Blood Pressure		Heart Rate (pulse per minute)	Notes (e.g. medication changes, activities)
		Systolic (upper #)	Diastolic (lower #)		
Monday	a.m.				
	a.m.				
	p.m.				
	p.m.				
Tuesday	a.m.				
	a.m.				
	p.m.				
	p.m.				
Wednesday	a.m.				
	a.m.				
	p.m.				
	p.m.				
Thursday	a.m.				
	a.m.				
	p.m.				
	p.m.				
Friday	a.m.				
	a.m.				
	p.m.				
	p.m.				
Saturday	a.m.				
	a.m.				
	p.m.				
	p.m.				
Sunday	a.m.				
	a.m.				
	p.m.				
	p.m.				

Blood Pressure Log

Month: ________________ **Week Starting:** __________________________

Time		Blood Pressure		Heart Rate (pulse per minute)	Notes (e.g. medication changes, activities)
		Systolic (upper #)	Diastolic (lower #)		
Monday	a.m.				
	a.m.				
	p.m.				
	p.m.				
Tuesday	a.m.				
	a.m.				
	p.m.				
	p.m.				
Wednesday	a.m.				
	a.m.				
	p.m.				
	p.m.				
Thursday	a.m.				
	a.m.				
	p.m.				
	p.m.				
Friday	a.m.				
	a.m.				
	p.m.				
	p.m.				
Saturday	a.m.				
	a.m.				
	p.m.				
	p.m.				
Sunday	a.m.				
	a.m.				
	p.m.				
	p.m.				

Blood Pressure Log

Month: ________________ **Week Starting:** __________________________

Time		Blood Pressure		Heart Rate (pulse per minute)	Notes (e.g. medication changes, activities)
		Systolic (upper #)	Diastolic (lower #)		
Monday	a.m.				
	a.m.				
	p.m.				
	p.m.				
Tuesday	a.m.				
	a.m.				
	p.m.				
	p.m.				
Wednesday	a.m.				
	a.m.				
	p.m.				
	p.m.				
Thursday	a.m.				
	a.m.				
	p.m.				
	p.m.				
Friday	a.m.				
	a.m.				
	p.m.				
	p.m.				
Saturday	a.m.				
	a.m.				
	p.m.				
	p.m.				
Sunday	a.m.				
	a.m.				
	p.m.				
	p.m.				

Blood Pressure Log

Month: ________________ **Week Starting:** ____________________________

Time		Blood Pressure		Heart Rate (pulse per minute)	Notes (e.g. medication changes, activities)
		Systolic (upper #)	Diastolic (lower #)		
Monday	a.m.				
	a.m.				
	p.m.				
	p.m.				
Tuesday	a.m.				
	a.m.				
	p.m.				
	p.m.				
Wednesday	a.m.				
	a.m.				
	p.m.				
	p.m.				
Thursday	a.m.				
	a.m.				
	p.m.				
	p.m.				
Friday	a.m.				
	a.m.				
	p.m.				
	p.m.				
Saturday	a.m.				
	a.m.				
	p.m.				
	p.m.				
Sunday	a.m.				
	a.m.				
	p.m.				
	p.m				

Blood Pressure Log

Month: ______________ **Week Starting:** ______________________

Time		Blood Pressure		Heart Rate (pulse per minute)	Notes (e.g. medication changes, activities)
		Systolic (upper #)	Diastolic (lower #)		
Monday	a.m.				
	a.m.				
	p.m.				
	p.m.				
Tuesday	a.m.				
	a.m.				
	p.m.				
	p.m.				
Wednesday	a.m.				
	a.m.				
	p.m.				
	p.m.				
Thursday	a.m.				
	a.m.				
	p.m.				
	p.m.				
Friday	a.m.				
	a.m.				
	p.m.				
	p.m.				
Saturday	a.m.				
	a.m.				
	p.m.				
	p.m.				
Sunday	a.m.				
	a.m.				
	p.m.				
	p.m.				

Blood Pressure Log

Month: ________________ **Week Starting:** _________________________

Time		Blood Pressure: Systolic (upper #)	Blood Pressure: Diastolic (lower #)	Heart Rate (pulse per minute)	Notes (e.g. medication changes, activities)
Monday	a.m.				
	a.m.				
	p.m.				
	p.m.				
Tuesday	a.m.				
	a.m.				
	p.m.				
	p.m.				
Wednesday	a.m.				
	a.m.				
	p.m.				
	p.m.				
Thursday	a.m.				
	a.m.				
	p.m.				
	p.m.				
Friday	a.m.				
	a.m.				
	p.m.				
	p.m.				
Saturday	a.m.				
	a.m.				
	p.m.				
	p.m.				
Sunday	a.m.				
	a.m.				
	p.m.				
	p.m.				

Blood Pressure Log

Month: ________________ Week Starting: ________________________

Time		Blood Pressure		Heart Rate (pulse per minute)	Notes (e.g. medication changes, activities)
		Systolic (upper #)	Diastolic (lower #)		
Monday	a.m.				
	a.m.				
	p.m.				
	p.m.				
Tuesday	a.m.				
	a.m.				
	p.m.				
	p.m.				
Wednesday	a.m.				
	a.m.				
	p.m.				
	p.m.				
Thursday	a.m.				
	a.m.				
	p.m.				
	p.m.				
Friday	a.m.				
	a.m.				
	p.m.				
	p.m.				
Saturday	a.m.				
	a.m.				
	p.m.				
	p.m.				
Sunday	a.m.				
	a.m.				
	p.m.				
	p.m.				

Blood Pressure Log

Month: ________________ **Week Starting:** __________________________

Time		Blood Pressure		Heart Rate (pulse per minute)	Notes (e.g. medication changes, activities)
		Systolic (upper #)	Diastolic (lower #)		
Monday	a.m.				
	a.m.				
	p.m.				
	p.m.				
Tuesday	a.m.				
	a.m.				
	p.m.				
	p.m.				
Wednesday	a.m.				
	a.m.				
	p.m.				
	p.m.				
Thursday	a.m.				
	a.m.				
	p.m.				
	p.m.				
Friday	a.m.				
	a.m.				
	p.m.				
	p.m.				
Saturday	a.m.				
	a.m.				
	p.m.				
	p.m.				
Sunday	a.m.				
	a.m.				
	p.m.				
	p.m.				

Blood Pressure Log

Month: ______________ **Week Starting:** ______________________

Time		Blood Pressure		Heart Rate (pulse per minute)	Notes (e.g. medication changes, activities)
		Systolic (upper #)	Diastolic (lower #)		
Monday	a.m.				
	a.m.				
	p.m.				
	p.m.				
Tuesday	a.m.				
	a.m.				
	p.m.				
	p.m.				
Wednesday	a.m.				
	a.m.				
	p.m.				
	p.m.				
Thursday	a.m.				
	a.m.				
	p.m.				
	p.m.				
Friday	a.m.				
	a.m.				
	p.m.				
	p.m.				
Saturday	a.m.				
	a.m.				
	p.m.				
	p.m.				
Sunday	a.m.				
	a.m.				
	p.m.				
	p.m.				

Blood Pressure Log

Month: ________________ **Week Starting:** ______________________

Time		Blood Pressure: Systolic (upper #)	Blood Pressure: Diastolic (lower #)	Heart Rate (pulse per minute)	Notes (e.g. medication changes, activities)
Monday	a.m.				
	a.m.				
	p.m.				
	p.m.				
Tuesday	a.m.				
	a.m.				
	p.m.				
	p.m.				
Wednesday	a.m.				
	a.m.				
	p.m.				
	p.m.				
Thursday	a.m.				
	a.m.				
	p.m.				
	p.m.				
Friday	a.m.				
	a.m.				
	p.m.				
	p.m.				
Saturday	a.m.				
	a.m.				
	p.m.				
	p.m.				
Sunday	a.m.				
	a.m.				
	p.m.				
	p.m.				

Blood Pressure Log

Month: _______________ Week Starting: _______________________

Time		Blood Pressure		Heart Rate (pulse per minute)	Notes (e.g. medication changes, activities)
		Systolic (upper #)	Diastolic (lower #)		
Monday	a.m.				
	a.m.				
	p.m.				
	p.m.				
Tuesday	a.m.				
	a.m.				
	p.m.				
	p.m.				
Wednesday	a.m.				
	a.m.				
	p.m.				
	p.m.				
Thursday	a.m.				
	a.m.				
	p.m.				
	p.m.				
Friday	a.m.				
	a.m.				
	p.m.				
	p.m.				
Saturday	a.m.				
	a.m.				
	p.m.				
	p.m.				
Sunday	a.m.				
	a.m.				
	p.m.				
	p.m.				

Blood Pressure Log

Month: ________________ **Week Starting:** ____________________________

Time		Blood Pressure		Heart Rate (pulse per minute)	Notes (e.g. medication changes, activities)
		Systolic (upper #)	**Diastolic** (lower #)		
Monday	a.m.				
	a.m.				
	p.m.				
	p.m.				
Tuesday	a.m.				
	a.m.				
	p.m.				
	p.m.				
Wednesday	a.m.				
	a.m.				
	p.m.				
	p.m.				
Thursday	a.m.				
	a.m.				
	p.m.				
	p.m.				
Friday	a.m.				
	a.m.				
	p.m.				
	p.m.				
Saturday	a.m.				
	a.m.				
	p.m.				
	p.m.				
Sunday	a.m.				
	a.m.				
	p.m.				
	p.m.				

Blood Pressure Log

Month: ________________ **Week Starting:** __________________________

Time		Blood Pressure		Heart Rate (pulse per minute)	Notes (e.g. medication changes, activities)
		Systolic (upper #)	Diastolic (lower #)		
Monday	a.m.				
	a.m.				
	p.m.				
	p.m.				
Tuesday	a.m.				
	a.m.				
	p.m.				
	p.m.				
Wednesday	a.m.				
	a.m.				
	p.m.				
	p.m.				
Thursday	a.m.				
	a.m.				
	p.m.				
	p.m.				
Friday	a.m.				
	a.m.				
	p.m.				
	p.m.				
Saturday	a.m.				
	a.m.				
	p.m.				
	p.m.				
Sunday	a.m.				
	a.m.				
	p.m.				
	p.m.				

Blood Pressure Log

Month: ________________ **Week Starting:** ____________________________

Time		Blood Pressure		Heart Rate (pulse per minute)	Notes (e.g. medication changes, activities)
		Systolic (upper #)	Diastolic (lower #)		
Monday	a.m.				
	a.m.				
	p.m.				
	p.m.				
Tuesday	a.m.				
	a.m.				
	p.m.				
	p.m.				
Wednesday	a.m.				
	a.m.				
	p.m.				
	p.m.				
Thursday	a.m.				
	a.m.				
	p.m.				
	p.m.				
Friday	a.m.				
	a.m.				
	p.m.				
	p.m.				
Saturday	a.m.				
	a.m.				
	p.m.				
	p.m.				
Sunday	a.m.				
	a.m.				
	p.m.				
	p.m.				

Blood Pressure Log

Month: ________________ **Week Starting:** _________________________

Time		Blood Pressure		Heart Rate (pulse per minute)	Notes (e.g. medication changes, activities)
		Systolic (upper #)	Diastolic (lower #)		
Monday	a.m.				
	a.m.				
	p.m.				
	p.m.				
Tuesday	a.m.				
	a.m.				
	p.m.				
	p.m.				
Wednesday	a.m.				
	a.m.				
	p.m.				
	p.m.				
Thursday	a.m.				
	a.m.				
	p.m.				
	p.m.				
Friday	a.m.				
	a.m.				
	p.m.				
	p.m.				
Saturday	a.m.				
	a.m.				
	p.m.				
	p.m.				
Sunday	a.m.				
	a.m.				
	p.m.				
	p.m.				

Blood Pressure Log

Month: _______________ **Week Starting:** _______________________

Time		Blood Pressure		Heart Rate (pulse per minute)	Notes (e.g. medication changes, activities)
		Systolic (upper #)	Diastolic (lower #)		
Monday	a.m.				
	a.m.				
	p.m.				
	p.m.				
Tuesday	a.m.				
	a.m.				
	p.m.				
	p.m.				
Wednesday	a.m.				
	a.m.				
	p.m.				
	p.m.				
Thursday	a.m.				
	a.m.				
	p.m.				
	p.m.				
Friday	a.m.				
	a.m.				
	p.m.				
	p.m.				
Saturday	a.m.				
	a.m.				
	p.m.				
	p.m.				
Sunday	a.m.				
	a.m.				
	p.m.				
	p.m.				

Blood Pressure Log

Month: ________________ **Week Starting:** _________________________

Time		Blood Pressure		Heart Rate (pulse per minute)	Notes (e.g. medication changes, activities)
		Systolic (upper #)	Diastolic (lower #)		
Monday	a.m.				
	a.m.				
	p.m.				
	p.m.				
Tuesday	a.m.				
	a.m.				
	p.m.				
	p.m.				
Wednesday	a.m.				
	a.m.				
	p.m.				
	p.m.				
Thursday	a.m.				
	a.m.				
	p.m.				
	p.m.				
Friday	a.m.				
	a.m.				
	p.m.				
	p.m.				
Saturday	a.m.				
	a.m.				
	p.m.				
	p.m.				
Sunday	a.m.				
	a.m.				
	p.m.				
	p.m.				

Blood Pressure Log

Month: ________________ **Week Starting:** __________________________

Time		Blood Pressure		Heart Rate (pulse per minute)	Notes (e.g. medication changes, activities)
		Systolic (upper #)	Diastolic (lower #)		
Monday	a.m.				
	a.m.				
	p.m.				
	p.m.				
Tuesday	a.m.				
	a.m.				
	p.m.				
	p.m.				
Wednesday	a.m.				
	a.m.				
	p.m.				
	p.m.				
Thursday	a.m.				
	a.m.				
	p.m.				
	p.m.				
Friday	a.m.				
	a.m.				
	p.m.				
	p.m.				
Saturday	a.m.				
	a.m.				
	p.m.				
	p.m.				
Sunday	a.m.				
	a.m.				
	p.m.				
	p.m.				

Blood Pressure Log

Month: ______________ Week Starting: ______________________

Time		Blood Pressure		Heart Rate (pulse per minute)	Notes (e.g. medication changes, activities)
		Systolic (upper #)	Diastolic (lower #)		
Monday	a.m.				
	a.m.				
	p.m.				
	p.m.				
Tuesday	a.m.				
	a.m.				
	p.m.				
	p.m.				
Wednesday	a.m.				
	a.m.				
	p.m.				
	p.m.				
Thursday	a.m.				
	a.m.				
	p.m.				
	p.m.				
Friday	a.m.				
	a.m.				
	p.m.				
	p.m.				
Saturday	a.m.				
	a.m.				
	p.m.				
	p.m.				
Sunday	a.m.				
	a.m.				
	p.m.				
	p.m.				

Blood Pressure Log

Month: _______________ **Week Starting:** ________________________

Time		Blood Pressure: Systolic (upper #)	Blood Pressure: Diastolic (lower #)	Heart Rate (pulse per minute)	Notes (e.g. medication changes, activities)
Monday	a.m.				
	a.m.				
	p.m.				
	p.m.				
Tuesday	a.m.				
	a.m.				
	p.m.				
	p.m.				
Wednesday	a.m.				
	a.m.				
	p.m.				
	p.m.				
Thursday	a.m.				
	a.m.				
	p.m.				
	p.m.				
Friday	a.m.				
	a.m.				
	p.m.				
	p.m.				
Saturday	a.m.				
	a.m.				
	p.m.				
	p.m.				
Sunday	a.m.				
	a.m.				
	p.m.				
	p.m.				

Blood Pressure Log

Month: ______________ **Week Starting:** ______________________

Time		Blood Pressure		Heart Rate (pulse per minute)	Notes (e.g. medication changes, activities)
		Systolic (upper #)	Diastolic (lower #)		
Monday	a.m.				
	a.m.				
	p.m.				
	p.m.				
Tuesday	a.m.				
	a.m.				
	p.m.				
	p.m.				
Wednesday	a.m.				
	a.m.				
	p.m.				
	p.m.				
Thursday	a.m.				
	a.m.				
	p.m.				
	p.m.				
Friday	a.m.				
	a.m.				
	p.m.				
	p.m.				
Saturday	a.m.				
	a.m.				
	p.m.				
	p.m.				
Sunday	a.m.				
	a.m.				
	p.m.				
	p.m.				

Blood Pressure Log

Month: ________________ **Week Starting:** ____________________________

Time		Blood Pressure: Systolic (upper #)	Blood Pressure: Diastolic (lower #)	Heart Rate (pulse per minute)	Notes (e.g. medication changes, activities)
Monday	a.m.				
	a.m.				
	p.m.				
	p.m.				
Tuesday	a.m.				
	a.m.				
	p.m.				
	p.m.				
Wednesday	a.m.				
	a.m.				
	p.m.				
	p.m.				
Thursday	a.m.				
	a.m.				
	p.m.				
	p.m.				
Friday	a.m.				
	a.m.				
	p.m.				
	p.m.				
Saturday	a.m.				
	a.m.				
	p.m.				
	p.m.				
Sunday	a.m.				
	a.m.				
	p.m.				
	p.m.				

Blood Pressure Log

Month: ________________ **Week Starting:** ________________________

Time		Blood Pressure: Systolic (upper #)	Blood Pressure: Diastolic (lower #)	Heart Rate (pulse per minute)	Notes (e.g. medication changes, activities)
Monday	a.m.				
	a.m.				
	p.m.				
	p.m.				
Tuesday	a.m.				
	a.m.				
	p.m.				
	p.m.				
Wednesday	a.m.				
	a.m.				
	p.m.				
	p.m.				
Thursday	a.m.				
	a.m.				
	p.m.				
	p.m.				
Friday	a.m.				
	a.m.				
	p.m.				
	p.m.				
Saturday	a.m.				
	a.m.				
	p.m.				
	p.m.				
Sunday	a.m.				
	a.m.				
	p.m.				
	p.m.				

Blood Pressure Log

Month: ________________ **Week Starting:** _________________________

Time		Blood Pressure: Systolic (upper #)	Blood Pressure: Diastolic (lower #)	Heart Rate (pulse per minute)	Notes (e.g. medication changes, activities)
Monday	a.m.				
	a.m.				
	p.m.				
	p.m.				
Tuesday	a.m.				
	a.m.				
	p.m.				
	p.m.				
Wednesday	a.m.				
	a.m.				
	p.m.				
	p.m.				
Thursday	a.m.				
	a.m.				
	p.m.				
	p.m.				
Friday	a.m.				
	a.m.				
	p.m.				
	p.m.				
Saturday	a.m.				
	a.m.				
	p.m.				
	p.m.				
Sunday	a.m.				
	a.m.				
	p.m.				
	p.m.				

Blood Pressure Log

Month: _______________ Week Starting: _______________________

Time		Blood Pressure		Heart Rate (pulse per minute)	Notes (e.g. medication changes, activities)
		Systolic (upper #)	Diastolic (lower #)		
Monday	a.m.				
	a.m.				
	p.m.				
	p.m.				
Tuesday	a.m.				
	a.m.				
	p.m.				
	p.m.				
Wednesday	a.m.				
	a.m.				
	p.m.				
	p.m.				
Thursday	a.m.				
	a.m.				
	p.m.				
	p.m.				
Friday	a.m.				
	a.m.				
	p.m.				
	p.m.				
Saturday	a.m.				
	a.m.				
	p.m.				
	p.m.				
Sunday	a.m.				
	a.m.				
	p.m.				
	p.m.				

Blood Pressure Log

Month: ________________ **Week Starting:** _________________________

Time		Blood Pressure		Heart Rate (pulse per minute)	Notes (e.g. medication changes, activities)
		Systolic (upper #)	Diastolic (lower #)		
Monday	a.m.				
	a.m.				
	p.m.				
	p.m.				
Tuesday	a.m.				
	a.m.				
	p.m.				
	p.m.				
Wednesday	a.m.				
	a.m.				
	p.m.				
	p.m.				
Thursday	a.m.				
	a.m.				
	p.m.				
	p.m.				
Friday	a.m.				
	a.m.				
	p.m.				
	p.m.				
Saturday	a.m.				
	a.m.				
	p.m.				
	p.m.				
Sunday	a.m.				
	a.m.				
	p.m.				
	p.m.				

Blood Pressure Log

Month: ______________ **Week Starting:** ________________________

Time		Blood Pressure		Heart Rate (pulse per minute)	Notes (e.g. medication changes, activities)
		Systolic (upper #)	Diastolic (lower #)		
Monday	a.m.				
	a.m.				
	p.m.				
	p.m.				
Tuesday	a.m.				
	a.m.				
	p.m.				
	p.m.				
Wednesday	a.m.				
	a.m.				
	p.m.				
	p.m.				
Thursday	a.m.				
	a.m.				
	p.m.				
	p.m.				
Friday	a.m.				
	a.m.				
	p.m.				
	p.m.				
Saturday	a.m.				
	a.m.				
	p.m.				
	p.m.				
Sunday	a.m.				
	a.m.				
	p.m.				
	p.m.				

Blood Pressure Log

Month: ________________ **Week Starting:** __________________________

Time		Blood Pressure: Systolic (upper #)	Blood Pressure: Diastolic (lower #)	Heart Rate (pulse per minute)	Notes (e.g. medication changes, activities)
Monday	a.m.				
	a.m.				
	p.m.				
	p.m.				
Tuesday	a.m.				
	a.m.				
	p.m.				
	p.m.				
Wednesday	a.m.				
	a.m.				
	p.m.				
	p.m.				
Thursday	a.m.				
	a.m.				
	p.m.				
	p.m.				
Friday	a.m.				
	a.m.				
	p.m.				
	p.m.				
Saturday	a.m.				
	a.m.				
	p.m.				
	p.m.				
Sunday	a.m.				
	a.m.				
	p.m.				
	p.m.				

Blood Pressure Log

Month: ________________ **Week Starting:** ____________________________

Time		Blood Pressure		Heart Rate (pulse per minute)	Notes (e.g. medication changes, activities)
		Systolic (upper #)	Diastolic (lower #)		
Monday	a.m.				
	a.m.				
	p.m.				
	p.m.				
Tuesday	a.m.				
	a.m.				
	p.m.				
	p.m.				
Wednesday	a.m.				
	a.m.				
	p.m.				
	p.m.				
Thursday	a.m.				
	a.m.				
	p.m.				
	p.m.				
Friday	a.m.				
	a.m.				
	p.m.				
	p.m.				
Saturday	a.m.				
	a.m.				
	p.m.				
	p.m.				
Sunday	a.m.				
	a.m.				
	p.m.				
	p.m.				

Blood Pressure Log

Month: ________________ Week Starting: _________________________

Time		Blood Pressure		Heart Rate (pulse per minute)	Notes (e.g. medication changes, activities)
		Systolic (upper #)	Diastolic (lower #)		
Monday	a.m.				
	a.m.				
	p.m.				
	p.m.				
Tuesday	a.m.				
	a.m.				
	p.m.				
	p.m.				
Wednesday	a.m.				
	a.m.				
	p.m.				
	p.m.				
Thursday	a.m.				
	a.m.				
	p.m.				
	p.m.				
Friday	a.m.				
	a.m.				
	p.m.				
	p.m.				
Saturday	a.m.				
	a.m.				
	p.m.				
	p.m.				
Sunday	a.m.				
	a.m.				
	p.m.				
	p.m.				

Blood Pressure Log

Month: ________________ **Week Starting:** ________________________

Time		Blood Pressure		Heart Rate (pulse per minute)	Notes (e.g. medication changes, activities)
		Systolic (upper #)	Diastolic (lower #)		
Monday	a.m.				
	a.m.				
	p.m.				
	p.m.				
Tuesday	a.m.				
	a.m.				
	p.m.				
	p.m.				
Wednesday	a.m.				
	a.m.				
	p.m.				
	p.m.				
Thursday	a.m.				
	a.m.				
	p.m.				
	p.m.				
Friday	a.m.				
	a.m.				
	p.m.				
	p.m.				
Saturday	a.m.				
	a.m.				
	p.m.				
	p.m.				
Sunday	a.m.				
	a.m.				
	p.m.				
	p.m.				

Blood Pressure Log

Month: ________________ **Week Starting**: ____________________________

Time		Blood Pressure		Heart Rate (pulse per minute)	Notes (e.g. medication changes, activities)
		Systolic (upper #)	Diastolic (lower #)		
Monday	a.m.				
	a.m.				
	p.m.				
	p.m.				
Tuesday	a.m.				
	a.m.				
	p.m.				
	p.m.				
Wednesday	a.m.				
	a.m.				
	p.m.				
	p.m.				
Thursday	a.m.				
	a.m.				
	p.m.				
	p.m.				
Friday	a.m.				
	a.m.				
	p.m.				
	p.m.				
Saturday	a.m.				
	a.m.				
	p.m.				
	p.m.				
Sunday	a.m.				
	a.m.				
	p.m.				
	p.m.				

Blood Pressure Log					

Month: ______________ Week Starting: ________________________

Time		Blood Pressure		Heart Rate (pulse per minute)	Notes (e.g. medication changes, activities)
		Systolic (upper #)	Diastolic (lower #)		
Monday	a.m.				
	a.m.				
	p.m.				
	p.m.				
Tuesday	a.m.				
	a.m.				
	p.m.				
	p.m.				
Wednesday	a.m.				
	a.m.				
	p.m.				
	p.m.				
Thursday	a.m.				
	a.m.				
	p.m.				
	p.m.				
Friday	a.m.				
	a.m.				
	p.m.				
	p.m.				
Saturday	a.m.				
	a.m.				
	p.m.				
	p.m.				
Sunday	a.m.				
	a.m.				
	p.m.				
	p.m.				

Blood Pressure Log

Month: ________________ **Week Starting:** __________________________

Time		Blood Pressure		Heart Rate (pulse per minute)	Notes (e.g. medication changes, activities)
		Systolic (upper #)	Diastolic (lower #)		
Monday	a.m.				
	a.m.				
	p.m.				
	p.m.				
Tuesday	a.m				
	a.m.				
	p.m.				
	p.m.				
Wednesday	a.m.				
	a.m.				
	p.m.				
	p.m.				
Thursday	a.m.				
	a.m.				
	p.m.				
	p.m.				
Friday	a.m.				
	a.m.				
	p.m.				
	p.m.				
Saturday	a.m.				
	a.m.				
	p.m.				
	p.m.				
Sunday	a.m.				
	a.m.				
	p.m.				
	p.m.				

Blood Pressure Log

Month: ______________ **Week Starting**: ______________________

Time		Blood Pressure		Heart Rate (pulse per minute)	Notes (e.g. medication changes, activities)
		Systolic (upper #)	Diastolic (lower #)		
Monday	a.m.				
	a.m.				
	p.m.				
	p.m.				
Tuesday	a.m.				
	a.m.				
	p.m.				
	p.m.				
Wednesday	a.m.				
	a.m.				
	p.m.				
	p.m.				
Thursday	a.m.				
	a.m.				
	p.m.				
	p.m.				
Friday	a.m.				
	a.m.				
	p.m.				
	p.m.				
Saturday	a.m.				
	a.m.				
	p.m.				
	p.m.				
Sunday	a.m.				
	a.m.				
	p.m.				
	p.m.				

Blood Pressure Log

Month: ________________ **Week Starting:** __________________________

Time		Blood Pressure		Heart Rate (pulse per minute)	Notes (e.g. medication changes, activities)
		Systolic (upper #)	Diastolic (lower #)		
Monday	a.m.				
	a.m.				
	p.m.				
	p.m.				
Tuesday	a.m.				
	a.m.				
	p.m.				
	p.m.				
Wednesday	a.m.				
	a.m.				
	p.m.				
	p.m.				
Thursday	a.m.				
	a.m.				
	p.m.				
	p.m.				
Friday	a.m.				
	a.m.				
	p.m.				
	p.m.				
Saturday	a.m.				
	a.m.				
	p.m.				
	p.m.				
Sunday	a.m.				
	a.m.				
	p.m.				
	p.m.				

Blood Pressure Log

Month: ________________ **Week Starting**: __________________________

Time		Blood Pressure		Heart Rate (pulse per minute)	Notes (e.g. medication changes, activities)
		Systolic (upper #)	Diastolic (lower #)		
Monday	a.m.				
	a.m.				
	p.m.				
	p.m.				
Tuesday	a.m.				
	a.m.				
	p.m.				
	p.m.				
Wednesday	a.m.				
	a.m.				
	p.m.				
	p.m.				
Thursday	a.m.				
	a.m.				
	p.m.				
	p.m.				
Friday	a.m.				
	a.m.				
	p.m.				
	p.m.				
Saturday	a.m.				
	a.m.				
	p.m.				
	p.m.				
Sunday	a.m.				
	a.m.				
	p.m.				
	p.m.				

Blood Pressure Log

Month: ________________ Week Starting: ___________________________

Time		Blood Pressure		Heart Rate (pulse per minute)	Notes (e.g. medication changes, activities)
		Systolic (upper #)	Diastolic (lower #)		
Monday	a.m.				
	a.m.				
	p.m.				
	p.m.				
Tuesday	a.m				
	a.m.				
	p.m.				
	p.m.				
Wednesday	a.m.				
	a.m.				
	p.m.				
	p.m.				
Thursday	a.m.				
	a.m.				
	p.m.				
	p.m.				
Friday	a.m.				
	a.m.				
	p.m.				
	p.m.				
Saturday	a.m.				
	a.m.				
	p.m.				
	p.m.				
Sunday	a.m.				
	a.m.				
	p.m.				
	p.m.				

Blood Pressure Log

Month: ______________ **Week Starting:** ________________________

Time		Blood Pressure		Heart Rate (pulse per minute)	Notes (e.g. medication changes, activities)
		Systolic (upper #)	Diastolic (lower #)		
Monday	a.m.				
	a.m.				
	p.m.				
	p.m.				
Tuesday	a.m.				
	a.m.				
	p.m.				
	p.m.				
Wednesday	a.m.				
	a.m.				
	p.m.				
	p.m.				
Thursday	a.m.				
	a.m.				
	p.m.				
	p.m.				
Friday	a.m.				
	a.m.				
	p.m.				
	p.m.				
Saturday	a.m.				
	a.m.				
	p.m.				
	p.m.				
Sunday	a.m.				
	a.m.				
	p.m.				
	p.m.				

Blood Pressure Log

Month: ________________ **Week Starting:** ______________________

Time		Blood Pressure		Heart Rate (pulse per minute)	Notes (e.g. medication changes, activities)
		Systolic (upper #)	Diastolic (lower #)		
Monday	a.m.				
	a.m.				
	p.m.				
	p.m.				
Tuesday	a.m.				
	a.m.				
	p.m.				
	p.m.				
Wednesday	a.m.				
	a.m.				
	p.m.				
	p.m.				
Thursday	a.m.				
	a.m.				
	p.m.				
	p.m.				
Friday	a.m.				
	a.m.				
	p.m.				
	p.m.				
Saturday	a.m.				
	a.m.				
	p.m.				
	p.m.				
Sunday	a.m.				
	a.m.				
	p.m.				
	p.m.				

Blood Pressure Log

Month: ________________ **Week Starting:** ____________________________

Time		Blood Pressure		Heart Rate (pulse per minute)	Notes (e.g. medication changes, activities)
		Systolic (upper #)	Diastolic (lower #)		
Monday	a.m.				
	a.m.				
	p.m.				
	p.m.				
Tuesday	a.m.				
	a.m.				
	p.m.				
	p.m.				
Wednesday	a.m.				
	a.m.				
	p.m.				
	p.m.				
Thursday	a.m.				
	a.m.				
	p.m.				
	p.m.				
Friday	a.m.				
	a.m.				
	p.m.				
	p.m.				
Saturday	a.m.				
	a.m.				
	p.m.				
	p.m.				
Sunday	a.m.				
	a.m.				
	p.m.				
	p.m.				

Blood Pressure Log					

Month: ________________ Week Starting: __________________________

Time		Blood Pressure		Heart Rate (pulse per minute)	Notes (e.g. medication changes, activities)
		Systolic (upper #)	Diastolic (lower #)		
Monday	a.m.				
	a.m.				
	p.m.				
	p.m.				
Tuesday	a.m.				
	a.m.				
	p.m.				
	p.m.				
Wednesday	a.m.				
	a.m.				
	p.m.				
	p.m.				
Thursday	a.m.				
	a.m.				
	p.m.				
	p.m.				
Friday	a.m.				
	a.m.				
	p.m.				
	p.m.				
Saturday	a.m.				
	a.m.				
	p.m.				
	p.m.				
Sunday	a.m.				
	a.m.				
	p.m.				
	p.m.				

Blood Pressure Log

Month: ________________ **Week Starting:** _________________________

Time		Blood Pressure		Heart Rate (pulse per minute)	Notes (e.g. medication changes, activities)
		Systolic (upper #)	Diastolic (lower #)		
Monday	a.m.				
	a.m.				
	p.m.				
	p.m.				
Tuesday	a.m.				
	a.m.				
	p.m.				
	p.m.				
Wednesday	a.m.				
	a.m.				
	p.m.				
	p.m.				
Thursday	a.m.				
	a.m.				
	p.m.				
	p.m.				
Friday	a.m.				
	a.m.				
	p.m.				
	p.m.				
Saturday	a.m.				
	a.m.				
	p.m.				
	p.m.				
Sunday	a.m.				
	a.m.				
	p.m.				
	p.m.				

Blood Pressure Log

Month: ________________ **Week Starting:** _________________________

Time		Blood Pressure: Systolic (upper #)	Blood Pressure: Diastolic (lower #)	Heart Rate (pulse per minute)	Notes (e.g. medication changes, activities)
Monday	a.m.				
	a.m.				
	p.m.				
	p.m.				
Tuesday	a.m				
	a.m.				
	p.m.				
	p.m.				
Wednesday	a.m.				
	a.m.				
	p.m.				
	p.m.				
Thursday	a.m.				
	a.m.				
	p.m.				
	p.m.				
Friday	a.m.				
	a.m.				
	p.m.				
	p.m.				
Saturday	a.m.				
	a.m.				
	p.m.				
	p.m.				
Sunday	a.m.				
	a.m.				
	p.m.				
	p.m.				

Blood Pressure Log

Month: _______________ **Week Starting:** ________________________

Time		Blood Pressure		Heart Rate (pulse per minute)	Notes (e.g. medication changes, activities)
		Systolic (upper #)	Diastolic (lower #)		
Monday	a.m.				
	a.m.				
	p.m.				
	p.m.				
Tuesday	a.m.				
	a.m.				
	p.m.				
	p.m.				
Wednesday	a.m.				
	a.m.				
	p.m.				
	p.m.				
Thursday	a.m.				
	a.m.				
	p.m.				
	p.m.				
Friday	a.m.				
	a.m.				
	p.m.				
	p.m.				
Saturday	a.m.				
	a.m.				
	p.m.				
	p.m.				
Sunday	a.m.				
	a.m.				
	p.m.				
	p.m.				

Blood Pressure Log

Month: ________________ Week Starting: __________________________

Time		Blood Pressure		Heart Rate (pulse per minute)	Notes (e.g. medication changes, activities)
		Systolic (upper #)	Diastolic (lower #)		
Monday	a.m.				
	a.m.				
	p.m.				
	p.m.				
Tuesday	a.m.				
	a.m.				
	p.m.				
	p.m.				
Wednesday	a.m.				
	a.m.				
	p.m.				
	p.m.				
Thursday	a.m.				
	a.m.				
	p.m.				
	p.m.				
Friday	a.m.				
	a.m.				
	p.m.				
	p.m.				
Saturday	a.m.				
	a.m.				
	p.m.				
	p.m.				
Sunday	a.m.				
	a.m.				
	p.m.				
	p.m.				

Blood Pressure Log

Month: ________________ **Week Starting:** __________________________

Time		Blood Pressure		Heart Rate (pulse per minute)	Notes (e.g. medication changes, activities)
		Systolic (upper #)	Diastolic (lower #)		
Monday	a.m.				
	a.m.				
	p.m.				
	p.m.				
Tuesday	a.m.				
	a.m.				
	p.m.				
	p.m.				
Wednesday	a.m.				
	a.m.				
	p.m.				
	p.m.				
Thursday	a.m.				
	a.m.				
	p.m.				
	p.m.				
Friday	a.m.				
	a.m.				
	p.m.				
	p.m.				
Saturday	a.m.				
	a.m.				
	p.m.				
	p.m.				
Sunday	a.m.				
	a.m.				
	p.m.				
	p.m.				

Blood Pressure Log

Month: ________________ Week Starting: ____________________________

Time		Blood Pressure		Heart Rate (pulse per minute)	Notes (e.g. medication changes, activities)
		Systolic (upper #)	Diastolic (lower #)		
Monday	a.m.				
	a.m.				
	p.m.				
	p.m.				
Tuesday	a.m.				
	a.m.				
	p.m.				
	p.m.				
Wednesday	a.m.				
	a.m.				
	p.m.				
	p.m.				
Thursday	a.m.				
	a.m.				
	p.m.				
	p.m.				
Friday	a.m.				
	a.m.				
	p.m.				
	p.m.				
Saturday	a.m.				
	a.m.				
	p.m.				
	p.m.				
Sunday	a.m.				
	a.m.				
	p.m.				
	p.m.				

Blood Pressure Log

Month: ________________ **Week Starting:** ___________________________

Time		Blood Pressure		Heart Rate (pulse per minute)	Notes (e.g. medication changes, activities)
		Systolic (upper #)	Diastolic (lower #)		
Monday	a.m.				
	a.m.				
	p.m.				
	p.m.				
Tuesday	a.m.				
	a.m.				
	p.m.				
	p.m.				
Wednesday	a.m.				
	a.m.				
	p.m.				
	p.m.				
Thursday	a.m.				
	a.m.				
	p.m.				
	p.m.				
Friday	a.m.				
	a.m.				
	p.m.				
	p.m.				
Saturday	a.m.				
	a.m.				
	p.m.				
	p.m.				
Sunday	a.m.				
	a.m.				
	p.m.				
	p.m.				

Blood Pressure Log

Month: ________________ **Week Starting**: __________________________

Time		Blood Pressure		Heart Rate (pulse per minute)	Notes (e.g. medication changes, activities)
		Systolic (upper #)	Diastolic (lower #)		
Monday	a.m.				
	a.m.				
	p.m.				
	p.m.				
Tuesday	a.m.				
	a.m.				
	p.m.				
	p.m.				
Wednesday	a.m.				
	a.m.				
	p.m.				
	p.m.				
Thursday	a.m.				
	a.m.				
	p.m.				
	p.m.				
Friday	a.m.				
	a.m.				
	p.m.				
	p.m.				
Saturday	a.m.				
	a.m.				
	p.m.				
	p.m.				
Sunday	a.m.				
	a.m.				
	p.m.				
	p.m.				

Blood Pressure Log

Month: ________________ **Week Starting:** __________________________

Time		Blood Pressure		Heart Rate (pulse per minute)	Notes (e.g. medication changes, activities)
		Systolic (upper #)	Diastolic (lower #)		
Monday	a.m.				
	a.m.				
	p.m.				
	p.m.				
Tuesday	a.m.				
	a.m.				
	p.m.				
	p.m.				
Wednesday	a.m.				
	a.m.				
	p.m.				
	p.m.				
Thursday	a.m.				
	a.m.				
	p.m.				
	p.m.				
Friday	a.m.				
	a.m.				
	p.m.				
	p.m.				
Saturday	a.m.				
	a.m.				
	p.m.				
	p.m.				
Sunday	a.m.				
	a.m.				
	p.m.				
	p.m.				

Blood Pressure Log

Month: ________________ **Week Starting:** __________________________

Time		Blood Pressure		Heart Rate (pulse per minute)	Notes (e.g. medication changes, activities)
		Systolic (upper #)	Diastolic (lower #)		
Monday	a.m.				
	a.m.				
	p.m.				
	p.m.				
Tuesday	a.m.				
	a.m.				
	p.m.				
	p.m.				
Wednesday	a.m.				
	a.m.				
	p.m.				
	p.m.				
Thursday	a.m.				
	a.m.				
	p.m.				
	p.m.				
Friday	a.m.				
	a.m.				
	p.m.				
	p.m.				
Saturday	a.m.				
	a.m.				
	p.m.				
	p.m.				
Sunday	a.m.				
	a.m.				
	p.m.				
	p.m.				

Blood Pressure Log

Month: ________________ Week Starting: __________________________

Time		Blood Pressure		Heart Rate (pulse per minute)	Notes (e.g. medication changes, activities)
		Systolic (upper #)	Diastolic (lower #)		
Monday	a.m.				
	a.m.				
	p.m.				
	p.m.				
Tuesday	a.m.				
	a.m.				
	p.m.				
	p.m.				
Wednesday	a.m.				
	a.m.				
	p.m.				
	p.m.				
Thursday	a.m.				
	a.m.				
	p.m.				
	p.m.				
Friday	a.m.				
	a.m.				
	p.m.				
	p.m.				
Saturday	a.m.				
	a.m.				
	p.m.				
	p.m.				
Sunday	a.m.				
	a.m.				
	p.m.				
	p.m.				

Blood Pressure Log

Month: ________________ Week Starting: __________________________

Time		Blood Pressure		Heart Rate (pulse per minute)	Notes (e.g. medication changes, activities)
		Systolic (upper #)	Diastolic (lower #)		
Monday	a.m.				
	a.m.				
	p.m.				
	p.m.				
Tuesday	a.m.				
	a.m.				
	p.m.				
	p.m.				
Wednesday	a.m.				
	a.m.				
	p.m.				
	p.m.				
Thursday	a.m.				
	a.m.				
	p.m.				
	p.m.				
Friday	a.m.				
	a.m.				
	p.m.				
	p.m.				
Saturday	a.m.				
	a.m.				
	p.m.				
	p.m.				
Sunday	a.m.				
	a.m.				
	p.m.				
	p.m.				

Blood Pressure Log

Month: ________________ **Week Starting:** ________________________

Time		Blood Pressure		Heart Rate (pulse per minute)	Notes (e.g. medication changes, activities)
		Systolic (upper #)	Diastolic (lower #)		
Monday	a.m.				
	a.m.				
	p.m.				
	p.m.				
Tuesday	a.m.				
	a.m.				
	p.m.				
	p.m.				
Wednesday	a.m.				
	a.m.				
	p.m.				
	p.m.				
Thursday	a.m.				
	a.m.				
	p.m.				
	p.m.				
Friday	a.m.				
	a.m.				
	p.m.				
	p.m.				
Saturday	a.m.				
	a.m.				
	p.m.				
	p.m.				
Sunday	a.m.				
	a.m.				
	p.m.				
	p.m.				

Blood Pressure Log

Month: ________________ Week Starting: ___________________________

Time		Blood Pressure		Heart Rate (pulse per minute)	Notes (e.g. medication changes, activities)
		Systolic (upper #)	Diastolic (lower #)		
Monday	a.m.				
	a.m.				
	p.m.				
	p.m.				
Tuesday	a.m.				
	a.m.				
	p.m.				
	p.m.				
Wednesday	a.m.				
	a.m.				
	p.m.				
	p.m.				
Thursday	a.m.				
	a.m.				
	p.m.				
	p.m.				
Friday	a.m.				
	a.m.				
	p.m.				
	p.m.				
Saturday	a.m.				
	a.m.				
	p.m.				
	p.m.				
Sunday	a.m.				
	a.m.				
	p.m.				
	p.m.				

Blood Pressure Log

Month: ________________ **Week Starting:** ____________________________

Time		Blood Pressure		Heart Rate (pulse per minute)	Notes (e.g. medication changes, activities)
		Systolic (upper #)	Diastolic (lower #)		
Monday	a.m.				
	a.m.				
	p.m.				
	p.m.				
Tuesday	a.m.				
	a.m.				
	p.m.				
	p.m.				
Wednesday	a.m.				
	a.m.				
	p.m.				
	p.m.				
Thursday	a.m.				
	a.m.				
	p.m.				
	p.m.				
Friday	a.m.				
	a.m.				
	p.m.				
	p.m.				
Saturday	a.m.				
	a.m.				
	p.m.				
	p.m.				
Sunday	a.m.				
	a.m.				
	p.m.				
	p.m.				

Blood Pressure Log

Month: ________________ **Week Starting:** __________________________

Time		Blood Pressure		Heart Rate (pulse per minute)	Notes (e.g. medication changes, activities)
		Systolic (upper #)	**Diastolic** (lower #)		
Monday	a.m.				
	a.m.				
	p.m.				
	p.m.				
Tuesday	a.m.				
	a.m.				
	p.m.				
	p.m.				
Wednesday	a.m.				
	a.m.				
	p.m.				
	p.m.				
Thursday	a.m.				
	a.m.				
	p.m.				
	p.m.				
Friday	a.m.				
	a.m.				
	p.m.				
	p.m.				
Saturday	a.m.				
	a.m.				
	p.m.				
	p.m.				
Sunday	a.m.				
	a.m.				
	p.m.				
	p.m.				

Blood Pressure Log

Month: ________________ **Week Starting**: ___________________________

Time		Blood Pressure		Heart Rate (pulse per minute)	Notes (e.g. medication changes, activities)
		Systolic (upper #)	Diastolic (lower #)		
Monday	a.m.				
	a.m.				
	p.m.				
	p.m.				
Tuesday	a.m.				
	a.m.				
	p.m.				
	p.m.				
Wednesday	a.m.				
	a.m.				
	p.m.				
	p.m.				
Thursday	a.m.				
	a.m.				
	p.m.				
	p.m.				
Friday	a.m.				
	a.m.				
	p.m.				
	p.m.				
Saturday	a.m.				
	a.m.				
	p.m.				
	p.m.				
Sunday	a.m.				
	a.m.				
	p.m.				
	p.m.				

Printed in Great Britain
by Amazon